Fitz Koehler

HEALTHY CANCER COMEBACK

journal

Fitzness Books

A division of Fitzness International LLC

Fitzness is a registered trademark of Fitz Koehler
and Fitzness International LLC
Gainesville, FL

For information or large orders, visit Fitzness.com
@Fitzness on Instagram, Facebook, and Youtube

Manufactured in the United States of America
Library of Congress Cataloging-in-Publication Data Available

Koehler, Fitz

Healthy Cancer Comeback: Journal

Fitzness International LLC non-fiction original paperback

1. Health & Fitness / Diseases & Conditions / Cancer
2. Self-Help – Journaling
3. Health & Fitness / Exercise / General

Cover Designer: Melissa Redon
Layout Designer: Melissa Redon
Proofreader: Jennifer Sen

ISBN 978-1-7355998-6-1

HeAltHy CaNCeR CoMebaCK
journal

Fitz Koehler, MSESS

My Fellow Cancer Crushers,

I hope this journal serves as a comforting and cathartic place to document your feelings, fears, friendships, joyful moments, and faith. Cancer is complicated, emotional, challenging, and loaded with unique experiences, but journaling has proven therapeutic effects and is a wise way to keep track of everything you're going through.

Share your laughter, tears, hopes, strange side effects, and "strawberry moments," which are the best parts of each day. Acknowledging good things as they happen will force much-needed joy into your life and foster an attitude of gratitude. Because even with cancer, silver linings can be abundant.

The back portion of this journal will allow you to use the knowledge you gained reading *Your Healthy Cancer Comeback: Sick to Strong* to set goals and document your path toward strength, stamina, vibrancy, and hopefully even athletic adventure.

I'm rooting for you!

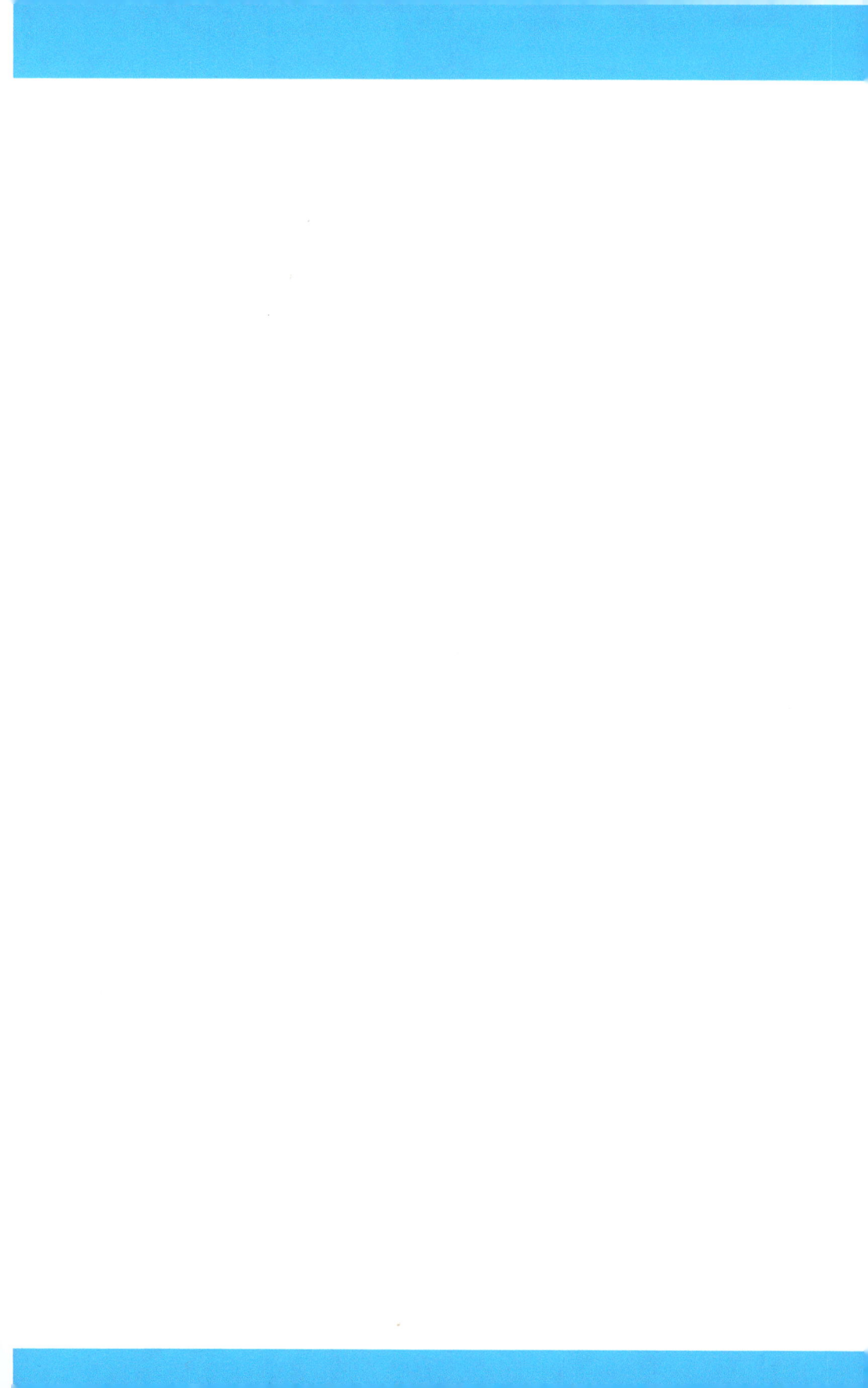

about me

MY NAME:

MY NICKNAME:

WHERE I LIVE:

MY AGE:

WHERE I WORK:

WHERE I GO TO SCHOOL:

MY FAMILY:

MY BFFS:

MY HOBBIES:

MY FITNESS STATUS:

WHAT I LOVE ABOUT ME:

my diagnosis:

This is how I discovered I might have cancer:

This is how I was told I definitely had cancer:

When I was diagnosed, I felt:

My treatment plan is as follows:

These are my doctors and my thoughts on each:

The cancer center I will be treated at:

My first day of treatment is:

My tentative last day of treatment will be:

The things that scare me most right now are:

The things that give me the most confidence are:

This is how I told my family, and these were their responses:

This is how I told my best friends, and these were their responses:

This is how I told my boss or colleagues, and these were their responses:

If you look for

a reason to smile,

you will find it!

I am grateful for...

I will pursue these passions no matter what:

The mantra I will repeat whenever things get particularly difficult:

I'm going to keep a positive attitude by focusing on:

My life is worth fighting for because...

10 things I'm committed to doing during treatment:

1

  2

3

  4

5

6

  7

   8

9

  10

10 things I can't wait to do when I'm done with treatment:

1

  2

3

  4

5

6

  7

  8

9

  10

The future me I'm striving to be:

My body will feel:

My body will be able to:

My body will look:

My attitude will be:

My work will be:

I will do these things for fun:

I will travel to:

My safe space to cry is:

I'm okay crying in front of:

I try hard not to cry in front of:

Crying makes me feel:

This makes me feel powerful:

This makes me feel normal:

This always makes me smile:

I feel most at peace when:

One thing I can not talk about:

One thing I wish I could talk about:

The thing I miss the most:

Things I do to distract myself from Cancer:

w°rk

How I've decided to handle my job during my treatment:

My experiences working through treatment:

I took time off from work during treatment and...

My colleagues have...

Getting dressed for work makes me:

Showing up to work during treatment makes me feel:

I've been working from home and...

How I feel about my job:

Someone at work I can confide in is:

Post-cancer, my career plans are:

Laugh at yourself
and everything else.
Cancer can be
ridiculous!

School

The school I'm attending:

The degree/certification I'm working towards:

How cancer is effecting my education:

Studying while undergoing treatment is:

How my teachers have responded:

My peers have been:

Learning during this process is:

I'm committed to:

My nutritional goals:

I will drink this much water daily:

I would like to eat more of these foods:

I would like to eat less of these foods:

I would like to drink less of this:

I would like to drink more of this:

A healthy food I would like to try is:

I would like to eat breakfast regularly because:

I would like to keep these snacks available to manage my hunger:

Meals I can plan and prepare ahead of time:

My favorite not-so-healthy indulgences:

My eXercise goals:

I'm going to exercise _____ days a week.

I want to try these three new activities:

1.

2.

3.

I want to be really good at this activity:

I would like to do this exercise in the water:

My favorite indoor exercises:

My favorite outdoor exercises:

My reasons for exercising alone:

My reasons for exercising in a group:

I could use an instructor or coach for:

I'm going to do independent research on this workout:

I would like to participate in this sport for leisure:

I would like to compete in this sport and win:

I would like to learn to:

Exercising with fellow cancer patients and survivors would be:

My sleep goals:

Lately, my sleep has been:

Things I'm doing to improve my quality of sleep:

I often dream about:

White noise is:

When I wake up, I feel:

My favorite place to sleep is:

My favorite person to cuddle with:

The most comfortable blanket I own is:

My perfect pillow is:

If I could change anything about my bedroom, it would be:

The thing I really love about my bedroom is:

The perfect way to say goodnight is:

zzzZZZ

My Appearance

I'm doing this to take care of my skin:

This is how I care for my lips:

My favorite cleanser:

The best moisturizer:

Since I started treatment, putting on makeup has been:

Why I love/hate to dress up now:

My favorite thing to wear:

I feel most attractive when:

This is what frustrates me about my appearance:

Meditation

This is where I prefer to meditate:

My technique for practicing meditation is:

Meditation makes me feel:

My Faith

Practicing my faith helps me:

Because of cancer, my commitment to my faith has:

I truly believe:

My Mental health

This is how I'm taking care of my mental health:

I need to do more of this to support my mental health:

I'm getting help from these forms of complementary care (examples: massage, physical therapy, acupuncture, counseling):

Cancer sucks, but it's brought these silver linings:

My caregivers,
what they do for me,
and why I love them:

When I'm done with cancer, I'm going to help others by:

My favorites

Favorite doctor:

Favorite nurse:

Favorite pet:

Favorite companions to go to appointments with:

Favorite books I'm reading:

Favorite cozy outfit:

Favorite blanket:

Favorite wig:

Favorite hat:

Favorite ways to relax:

Favorite ways to vent frustrations:

.

Favorite ways to have fun:

Nicknames

for my port:

for my tumor:

for my ostomy bag:

for my bald head:

for my doctors:

for my nurses:

for my caregiver:

for me and my changing appearance:

Draw your port as a cartoon character with a face, body, and clothes:

Chemo

My treatment plan for chemo is:

The drugs I will be receiving:

Chemo makes me feel:

Side effects:

Solutions for my side-effects:

Chemo makes everything taste:

These are my go-to foods when my stomach and taste buds go on strike:

The vibe of the room where I get chemo:

Seeing other patients makes me feel:

My relationship with needles:

This is how I kill time during chemo:

Someone interesting I met while getting chemo:

Something I actually like about the chemo experience is:

Chemo Countdown

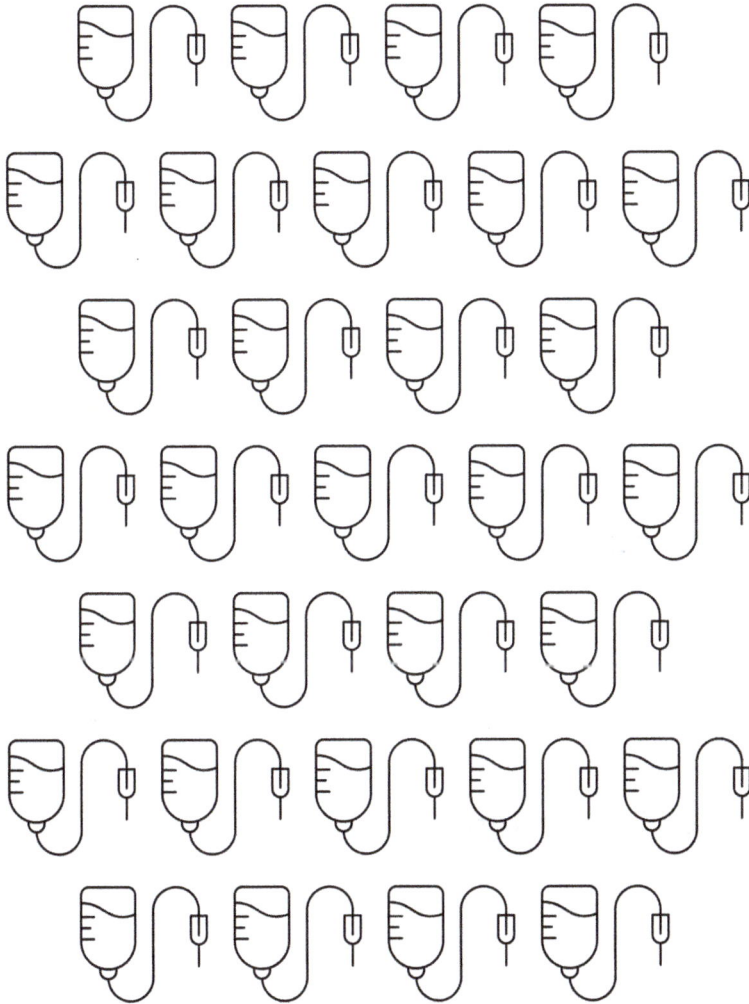

My bald head

The most surprising part:

The best part:

The worst part:

When I look in the mirror, I think:

Wigs or No Wigs? Why?:

When my hair grows back, I will:

My bald head makes me look like this celebrity:

DECORATE THE HEAD

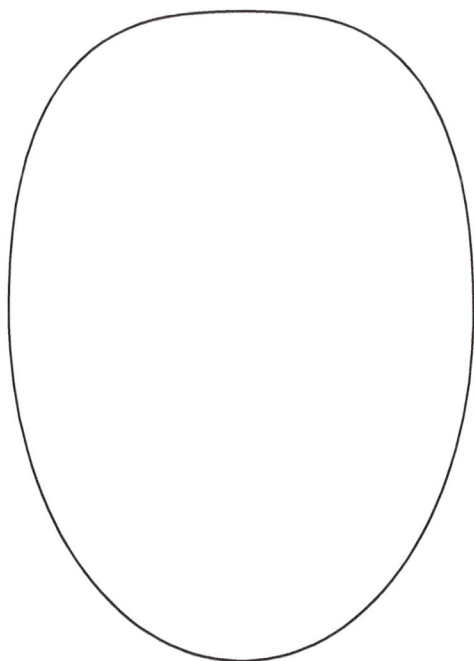

Radiation

My treatment plan for radiation is:

Getting zapped makes me feel:

I do this to prevent burns:

The process of getting zapped is:

Side effects:

Solutions for my side effects:

Sommeone interesting I met at my radiation appointment is:

Something I actually like about the radiation experience is:

Radiation Countdown

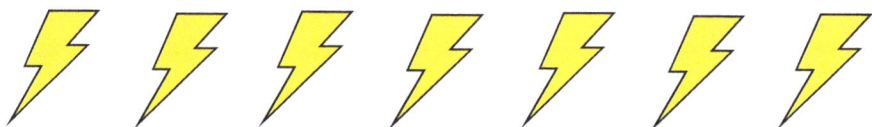

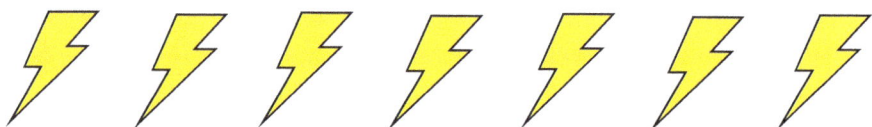

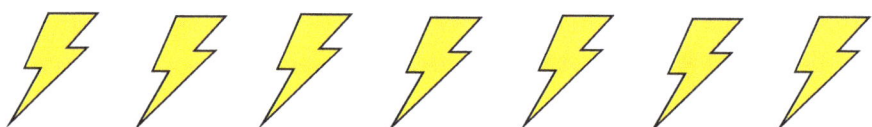

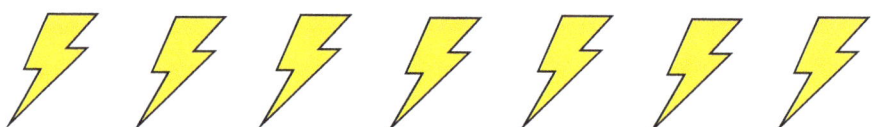

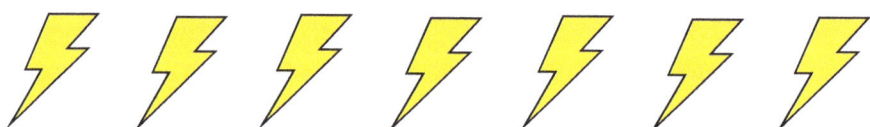

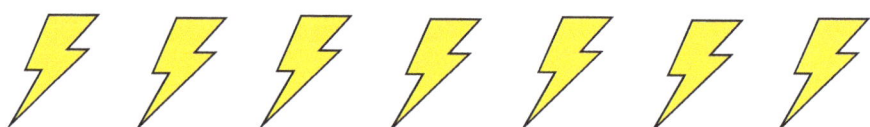

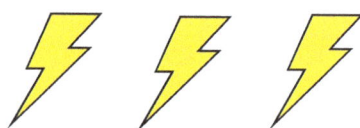

Perspective

is

powerful.

Surgery

Type of surgery/surgeries I'm having:

Where I'm having surgery:

My surgeon is:

The bright side of surgery:

The worst part of the surgery:

This is my recovery plan:

Someone interesting I've met because of surgery:

Surgery has changed my body:

My changed body makes me feel:

Surgery Countdown

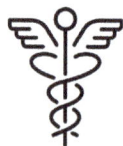

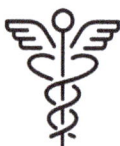

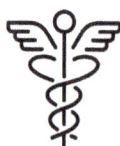

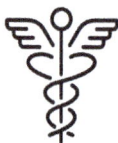

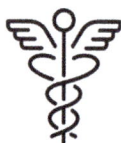

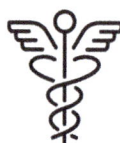

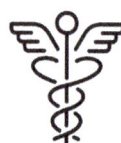

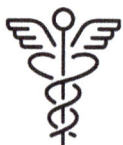

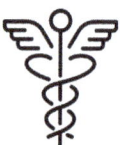

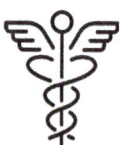

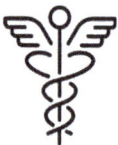

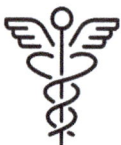

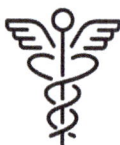

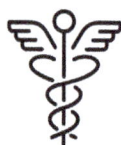

Show

compassion

for you!

Transplants and Implants

I've had this removed:

This will be my replacement:

These surgeries make me feel:

I'm nervous because:

I'm grateful because:

I'm confident because:

Life after the transplant/implant will be:

The story of my transplant goes like this ...

Five words to describe each of my doctors:

If I had to rank my cancer treatments from best to worst...

This experience was really traumatic:

My medicine cabinet looks like:

Questions I need to ask at my next appointment:

My five favorite public restrooms and why:

1

2

3

4

5

Control

what you

can.

fitness favorites

My favorite types of cardio:

My favorite strength training exercises:

My favorite body parts to stretch:

My favorite balance training exercises:

My favorite indoor places to exercise:

My favorite places to walk/hike:

My favorite things to do outside:

Pamper yourself

whenever possible.

CaNCAN awards

Best friend to vent to:

Favorite shoulder to cry on:

Most brilliant pal to discuss cancer with:

Best hugger:

Most likely to make me laugh:

Most helpful neighbor:

Best phone friend:

Most helpful family members:

Friend who sends the best text messages:

Most helpful coworkers:

Most lovable pet:

Most thoughtful gifts have been:

Special cards I've received:

Favorite place to mentally escape:

Favorite uplifting song:

Favorite podcast:

Favorite shows to binge on rest days:

Favorite musical artist:

Favorite comedian:

Favorite book:

Favorite movie:

Favorite play:

Celebrity I'm crushing on:

Favorite doctor:

Favorite nurse:

Favorite way to have fun:

You can do

hard things!

Cranky Files

These people made my life more difficult:

I hate these drugs so much:

Worst side-effects in the world:

136

My least favorite medical professional:

The worst thing I've been forced to drink:

I loath having this exam:

I wish my body would stop:

I wish my body would start:

When I'm cranky I want to:

Exercise and nutrition can make your body a hostile home for cancer!

favorite ways to say F*ck cancer

Strangest and most awkward things people have said to me

This is how I'd really like to respond to some of those strange statements:

Kind things strangers have said to me or done for me

So Famous

The title of the book about my life would be...

If my life were a TV show, this would be the theme song...

The celebrity who would play the role of ME is:

My catchphrase would be:

Enjoy the rain

on your

bald head.

I'm going to help
find a cure for my
disease by...

songs that inspire me

shows I'm planning on binge-watching

things that make me laugh

my role mOdels are...

I hope these people know how much they mean to me

(Write names and reasons)

Scan Log

Scan Type:

Date:

Results:

Scan Type:

Date:

Results:

Scan Type:

Date:

Results:

Scan Log

Scan Type:

Date:

Results:

Scan Type:

Date:

Results:

Scan Type:

Date:

Results:

Scan Log

Scan Type:

Date:

Results:

Scan Type:

Date:

Results:

Scan Type:

Date:

Results:

Scan Log

Scan Type:

Date:

Results:

Scan Type:

Date:

Results:

Scan Type:

Date:

Results:

weekly weight check-ins

My healthy weight is:

Week-by-week weight changes

Date:

Weight:

Date:

Weight:

Date:

Weight:

Date:

Weight:

Date:

Weight:

Date:

Weight:

Date:

Weight:

Date:

Weight:

Date:

Weight:

Date:

Weight:

Date: Date:

Weight: Weight:

Date: Date:

Weight: Weight:

Date: Date:

Weight: Weight:

Date: Date:

Weight: Weight:

Date: Date:

Weight: Weight:

Date: Date:

Weight: Weight:

Date: Date:

Weight: Weight:

Date: Date:

Weight: Weight:

Date: Date:

Weight: Weight:

Date: Date:

Weight: Weight:

Date: Date:

Weight: Weight:

Date: Date:

Weight: Weight:

Date: Date:

Weight: Weight:

Date: Date:

Weight: Weight:

Date: Date:

Weight: Weight:

Date: Date:

Weight: Weight:

Date: Date:

Weight: Weight:

Date: Date:

Weight: Weight:

Date: Date:

Weight: Weight:

Date: Date:

Weight: Weight:

Date: Date:

Weight: Weight:

Date: Date:

Weight: Weight:

Date: Date:

Weight: Weight:

Choose strength

over weakness!

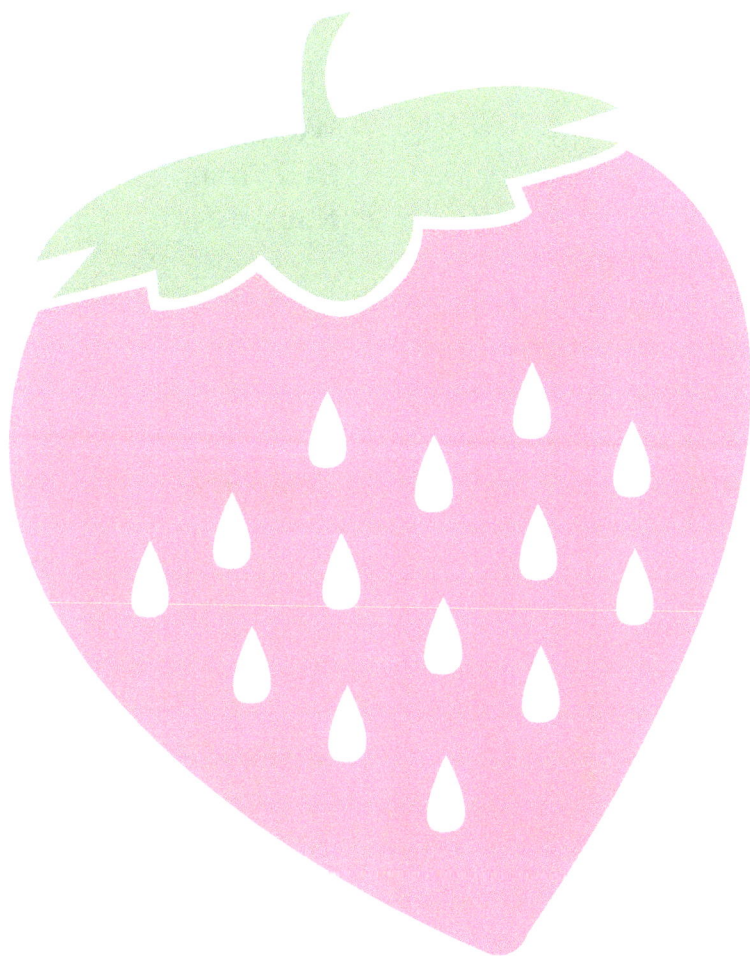

Strawberry Moments

Acknowledge the sweetest parts of each day by writing down your strawberry moments. Focusing on the silver linings in this weird world of cancer can lift your spirits and help you maintain perspective.

Daily jOurnal

DAY / DATE :

SLEEP
Wake up Time:
Bed Time:
Naps:

ENERGY LEVEL :

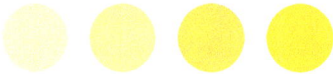

EXERCISE :

Strength	Flexibility

Cardio	Balance

MY DAILY EXERCISE RATED :

TODAY'S WATER
CONSUMPTION :

THREE HEALTHY
FOODS I ATE TODAY:

1

2

3

I conquered this hard thing today:

Strawberry moments:

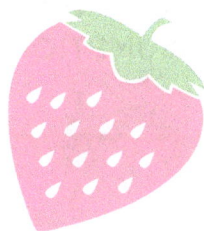

Daily jOurnal

DAY / DATE :

SLEEP
Wake up Time:
Bed Time:
Naps:

ENERGY LEVEL :

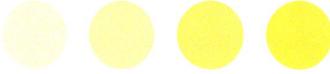

EXERCISE :

Strength	Flexibility

Cardio	Balance

MY DAILY EXERCISE RATED :

TODAY'S WATER
CONSUMPTION :

THREE HEALTHY
FOODS I ATE TODAY:

1

2

3

I conquered this hard thing today:

Strawberry moments:

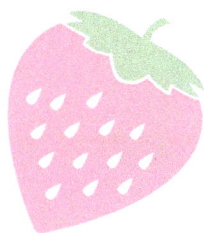

Daily jOurnal

DAY / DATE :

SLEEP
Wake up Time:
Bed Time:
Naps:

ENERGY LEVEL :

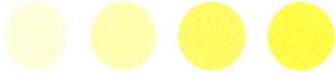

EXERCISE :

Strength	Flexibility

Cardio	Balance

MY DAILY EXERCISE RATED :

THREE HEALTHY
FOODS I ATE TODAY:

1

TODAY'S WATER
CONSUMPTION :

2

3

I conquered this hard thing today:

Strawberry moments:

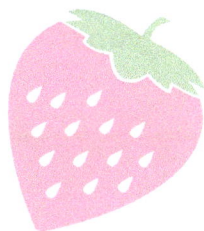

Daily journal

DAY / DATE :

SLEEP
Wake up Time:
Bed Time:
Naps:

ENERGY LEVEL :

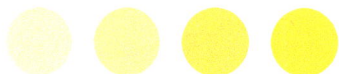

EXERCISE :

Strength	Flexibility

Cardio	Balance

MY DAILY EXERCISE RATED :

THREE HEALTHY
FOODS I ATE TODAY:

TODAY'S WATER
CONSUMPTION :

1

2

3

I conquered this hard thing today:

Strawberry moments:

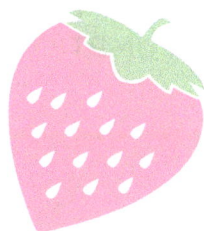

Daily jOurnal

DAY / DATE :

SLEEP
Wake up Time:
Bed Time:
Naps:

ENERGY LEVEL :

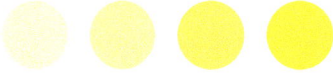

EXERCISE :

Strength	Flexibility
Cardio	**Balance**

MY DAILY EXERCISE RATED :

TODAY'S WATER
CONSUMPTION :

THREE HEALTHY
FOODS I ATE TODAY:

1

2

3

I conquered this hard thing today:

Strawberry moments:

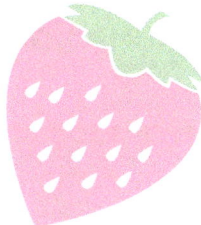

Daily jOurnal

DAY / DATE :

SLEEP
Wake up Time:
Bed Time:
Naps:

ENERGY LEVEL :

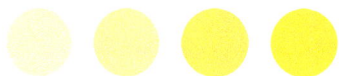

EXERCISE :

Strength	Flexibility

Cardio	Balance

MY DAILY EXERCISE RATED :

THREE HEALTHY
FOODS I ATE TODAY:

TODAY'S WATER
CONSUMPTION :

1

2

3

I conquered this hard thing today:

Strawberry moments:

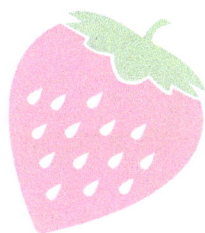

Daily jOurnal

DAY / DATE :

SLEEP
Wake up Time:
Bed Time:
Naps:

ENERGY LEVEL :

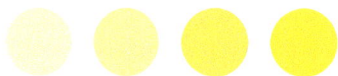

EXERCISE :

Strength	Flexibility

Cardio	Balance

MY DAILY EXERCISE RATED :

TODAY'S WATER
CONSUMPTION :

THREE HEALTHY
FOODS I ATE TODAY:

1

2

3

I conquered this hard thing today:

Strawberry moments:

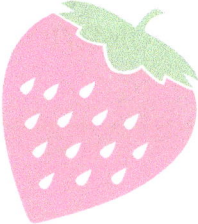

Daily jOurnal

DAY / DATE :

SLEEP
Wake up Time:
Bed Time:
Naps:

ENERGY LEVEL :

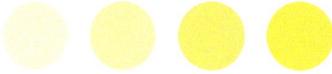

EXERCISE :

Strength	Flexibility

Cardio	Balance

MY DAILY EXERCISE RATED :

THREE HEALTHY FOODS I ATE TODAY:

1

2

3

TODAY'S WATER CONSUMPTION :

I conquered this hard thing today:

Strawberry moments:

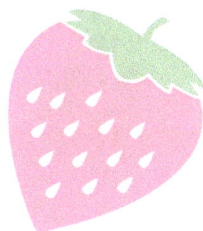

Daily jOurnal

DAY / DATE :

SLEEP
Wake up Time:
Bed Time:
Naps:

ENERGY LEVEL :

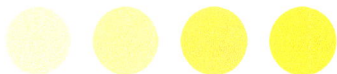

EXERCISE :

Strength	Flexibility
Cardio	Balance

MY DAILY EXERCISE RATED :

TODAY'S WATER
CONSUMPTION :

THREE HEALTHY
FOODS I ATE TODAY:

1

2

3

I conquered this hard thing today:

Strawberry moments:

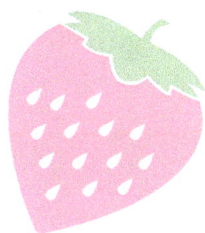

Daily jOurnal

DAY / DATE :

SLEEP
Wake up Time:
Bed Time:
Naps:

ENERGY LEVEL :

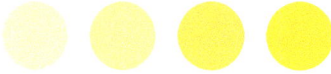

EXERCISE :

Strength	Flexibility
Cardio	Balance

MY DAILY EXERCISE RATED :

THREE HEALTHY
FOODS I ATE TODAY:

1

TODAY'S WATER
CONSUMPTION :

2

3

I conquered this hard thing today:

Strawberry moments:

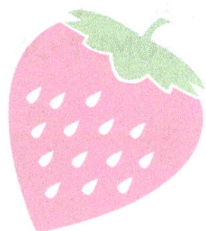

Daily jOurnal

DAY / DATE :

SLEEP
Wake up Time:
Bed Time:
Naps:

ENERGY LEVEL :

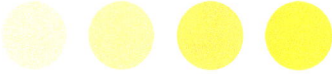

EXERCISE :

Strength	Flexibility

Cardio	Balance

MY DAILY EXERCISE RATED :

THREE HEALTHY FOODS I ATE TODAY:

1

TODAY'S WATER CONSUMPTION :

2

3

I conquered this hard thing today:

Strawberry moments:

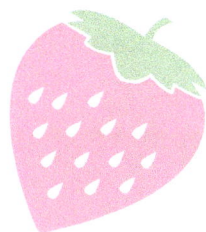

Daily jOurnal

DAY / DATE :

SLEEP
Wake up Time:
Bed Time:
Naps:

ENERGY LEVEL :

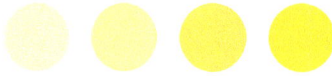

EXERCISE :

Strength	Flexibility

Cardio	Balance

MY DAILY EXERCISE RATED :

THREE HEALTHY FOODS I ATE TODAY:

TODAY'S WATER CONSUMPTION :

1

2

3

I conquered this hard thing today:

Strawberry moments:

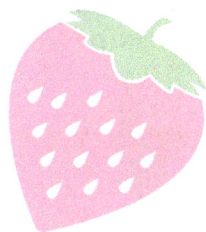

Daily jOurnal

DAY / DATE :

SLEEP
Wake up Time:
Bed Time:
Naps:

ENERGY LEVEL :

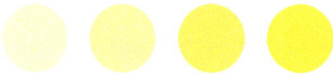

EXERCISE :

Strength	Flexibility

Cardio	Balance

MY DAILY EXERCISE RATED :

THREE HEALTHY
FOODS I ATE TODAY:

TODAY'S WATER
CONSUMPTION :

1

2

3

I conquered this hard thing today:

Strawberry moments:

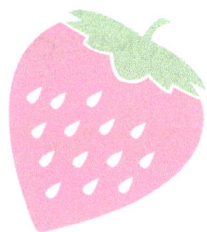

Daily journal

DAY / DATE :

SLEEP
Wake up Time:
Bed Time:
Naps:

ENERGY LEVEL :

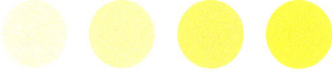

EXERCISE :

Strength	Flexibility

Cardio	Balance

MY DAILY EXERCISE RATED :

THREE HEALTHY FOODS I ATE TODAY:

1

TODAY'S WATER CONSUMPTION :

2

3

I conquered this hard thing today:

Strawberry moments:

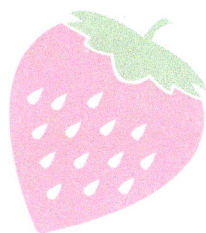

Daily jOurnal

DAY / DATE :

SLEEP
Wake up Time:
Bed Time:
Naps:

ENERGY LEVEL :

EXERCISE :

Strength	Flexibility

Cardio	Balance

MY DAILY EXERCISE RATED :

THREE HEALTHY FOODS I ATE TODAY:

TODAY'S WATER CONSUMPTION :

1

2

3

I conquered this hard thing today:

Strawberry moments:

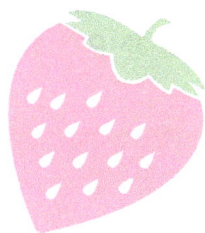

Daily jOurnal

DAY / DATE :

SLEEP
Wake up Time:
Bed Time:
Naps:

ENERGY LEVEL :

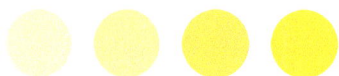

EXERCISE :

Strength	Flexibility

Cardio	Balance

MY DAILY EXERCISE RATED :

THREE HEALTHY
FOODS I ATE TODAY:

TODAY'S WATER
CONSUMPTION :

1

2

3

I conquered this hard thing today:

Strawberry moments:

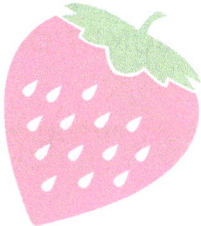

Daily jOurnal

DAY / DATE :

SLEEP
Wake up Time:
Bed Time:
Naps:

ENERGY LEVEL :

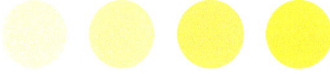

EXERCISE :

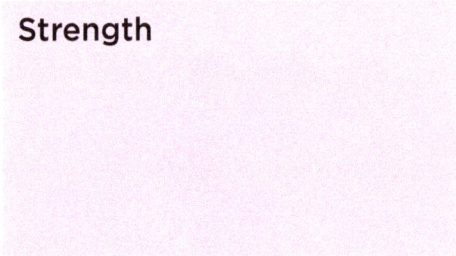
Strength

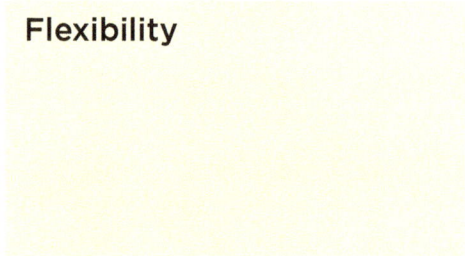
Flexibility

Cardio

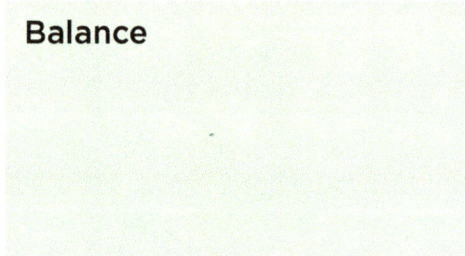
Balance

MY DAILY EXERCISE RATED :

THREE HEALTHY FOODS I ATE TODAY:

1

2

3

TODAY'S WATER CONSUMPTION :

I conquered this hard thing today:

Strawberry moments:

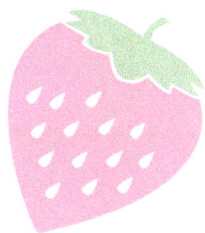

Daily jOurnal

DAY / DATE :

SLEEP
Wake up Time:
Bed Time:
Naps:

ENERGY LEVEL :

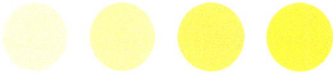

EXERCISE :

Strength	Flexibility

Cardio	Balance

MY DAILY EXERCISE RATED :

TODAY'S WATER
CONSUMPTION :

THREE HEALTHY
FOODS I ATE TODAY:

1

2

3

I conquered this hard thing today:

Strawberry moments:

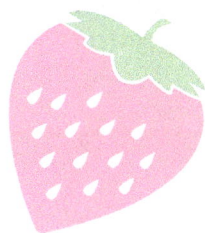

Daily jOurnal

DAY / DATE :

SLEEP
Wake up Time:
Bed Time:
Naps:

ENERGY LEVEL :

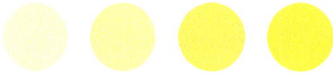

EXERCISE :

Strength	**Flexibility**

Cardio	**Balance**

MY DAILY EXERCISE RATED :

TODAY'S WATER
CONSUMPTION :

THREE HEALTHY
FOODS I ATE TODAY:

1

2

3

I conquered this hard thing today:

Strawberry moments:

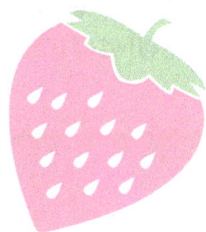

Daily jOurnal

DAY / DATE :

SLEEP
Wake up Time:
Bed Time:
Naps:

ENERGY LEVEL :

EXERCISE :

Strength	Flexibility

Cardio	Balance

MY DAILY EXERCISE RATED :

TODAY'S WATER CONSUMPTION :

THREE HEALTHY FOODS I ATE TODAY:

1

2

3

I conquered this hard thing today:

Strawberry moments:

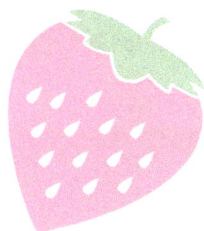

Daily jOurnal

DAY / DATE :

SLEEP
Wake up Time:
Bed Time:
Naps:

ENERGY LEVEL :

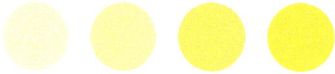

EXERCISE :

Strength	Flexibility

Cardio	Balance

MY DAILY EXERCISE RATED :

TODAY'S WATER
CONSUMPTION :

THREE HEALTHY
FOODS I ATE TODAY:

1

2

3

I conquered this hard thing today:

Strawberry moments:

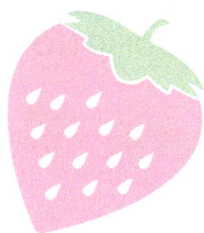

Daily jOurnal

DAY / DATE :

SLEEP
Wake up Time:
Bed Time:
Naps:

ENERGY LEVEL :

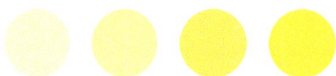

EXERCISE :

Strength	Flexibility

Cardio	Balance

MY DAILY EXERCISE RATED :

TODAY'S WATER
CONSUMPTION :

THREE HEALTHY
FOODS I ATE TODAY:

1

2

3

I conquered this hard thing today:

Strawberry moments:

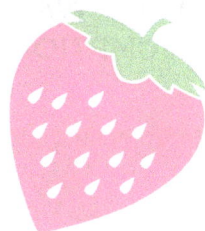

Daily jOurnal

DAY / DATE :

SLEEP
Wake up Time:
Bed Time:
Naps:

ENERGY LEVEL :

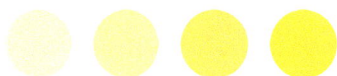

EXERCISE :

Strength	Flexibility

Cardio	Balance

MY DAILY EXERCISE RATED :

THREE HEALTHY FOODS I ATE TODAY:

1

2

3

TODAY'S WATER CONSUMPTION :

I conquered this hard thing today:

Strawberry moments:

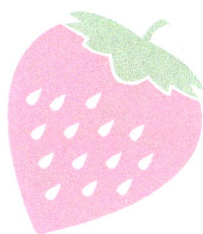

Daily jOurnal

DAY / DATE :

SLEEP
Wake up Time:
Bed Time:
Naps:

ENERGY LEVEL :

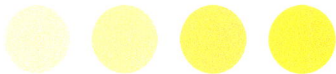

EXERCISE :

| Strength | Flexibility |

| Cardio | Balance |

MY DAILY EXERCISE RATED :

TODAY'S WATER CONSUMPTION :

THREE HEALTHY FOODS I ATE TODAY:

1

2

3

I conquered this hard thing today:

Strawberry moments:

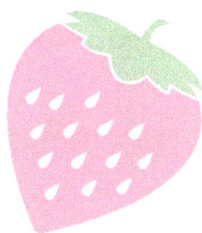

Daily jOurnal

DAY / DATE :

SLEEP
Wake up Time:
Bed Time:
Naps:

ENERGY LEVEL :

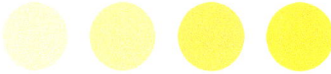

EXERCISE :

Strength	Flexibility

Cardio	Balance

MY DAILY EXERCISE RATED :

TODAY'S WATER
CONSUMPTION :

THREE HEALTHY
FOODS I ATE TODAY:

1

2

3

I conquered this hard thing today:

Strawberry moments:

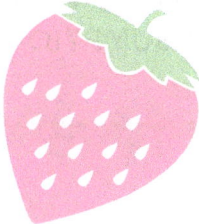

Daily jOurnal

DAY / DATE :

SLEEP
Wake up Time:
Bed Time:
Naps:

ENERGY LEVEL :

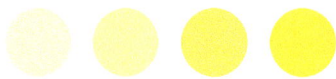

EXERCISE :

Strength	Flexibility
Cardio	Balance

MY DAILY EXERCISE RATED :

THREE HEALTHY
FOODS I ATE TODAY:

1

TODAY'S WATER
CONSUMPTION :

2

3

I conquered this hard thing today:

Strawberry moments:

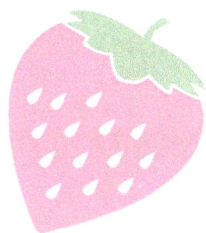

Daily jOurnal

DAY / DATE :

SLEEP
Wake up Time:
Bed Time:
Naps:

ENERGY LEVEL :

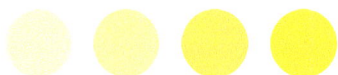

EXERCISE :

Strength	Flexibility
Cardio	Balance

MY DAILY EXERCISE RATED :

THREE HEALTHY
FOODS I ATE TODAY:

TODAY'S WATER
CONSUMPTION :

1

2

3

I conquered this hard thing today:

Strawberry moments:

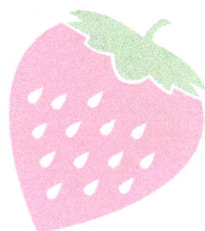

Daily jOurnal

DAY / DATE :

SLEEP
Wake up Time:
Bed Time:
Naps:

ENERGY LEVEL :

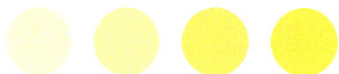

EXERCISE :

Strength	Flexibility

Cardio	Balance

MY DAILY EXERCISE RATED :

THREE HEALTHY FOODS I ATE TODAY:

1

TODAY'S WATER CONSUMPTION :

2

3

I conquered this hard thing today:

Strawberry moments:

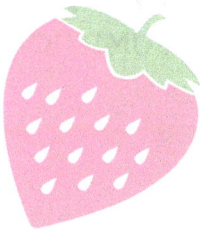

Daily jOurnal

DAY / DATE :

SLEEP
Wake up Time:
Bed Time:
Naps:

ENERGY LEVEL :

EXERCISE :

Strength	Flexibility

Cardio	Balance

MY DAILY EXERCISE RATED :

THREE HEALTHY
FOODS I ATE TODAY:

TODAY'S WATER
CONSUMPTION :

1

2

3

I conquered this hard thing today:

Strawberry moments:

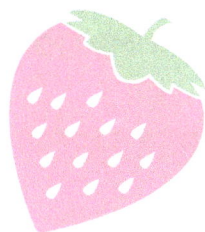

Daily jOurnal

DAY / DATE :

SLEEP
Wake up Time:
Bed Time:
Naps:

ENERGY LEVEL :

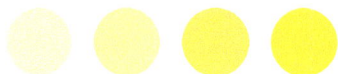

EXERCISE :

Strength	Flexibility

Cardio	Balance

MY DAILY EXERCISE RATED :

TODAY'S WATER
CONSUMPTION :

THREE HEALTHY
FOODS I ATE TODAY:

1

2

3

I conquered this hard thing today:

Strawberry moments:

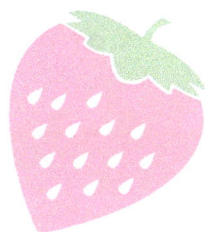

Daily jOurnal

DAY / DATE :

SLEEP
Wake up Time:
Bed Time:
Naps:

ENERGY LEVEL :

EXERCISE :

Strength	Flexibility

Cardio	Balance

MY DAILY EXERCISE RATED :

THREE HEALTHY
FOODS I ATE TODAY:

TODAY'S WATER
CONSUMPTION :

1

2

3

I conquered this hard thing today:

Strawberry moments:

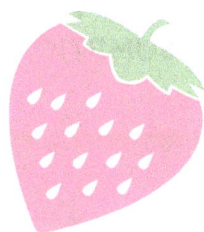

Daily jOurnal

DAY / DATE :

SLEEP
Wake up Time:
Bed Time:
Naps:

ENERGY LEVEL :

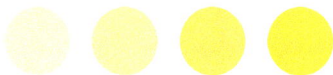

EXERCISE :

Strength	Flexibility

Cardio	Balance

MY DAILY EXERCISE RATED :

THREE HEALTHY
FOODS I ATE TODAY:

TODAY'S WATER
CONSUMPTION :

1

2

3

I conquered this hard thing today:

Strawberry moments:

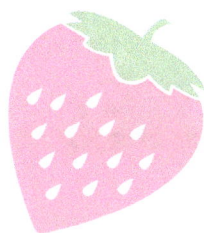

Daily jOurnal

DAY / DATE :

SLEEP
Wake up Time:
Bed Time:
Naps:

ENERGY LEVEL :

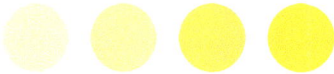

EXERCISE :

Strength	Flexibility
Cardio	Balance

MY DAILY EXERCISE RATED :

THREE HEALTHY
FOODS I ATE TODAY:

TODAY'S WATER
CONSUMPTION :

1

2

3

I conquered this hard thing today:

Strawberry moments:

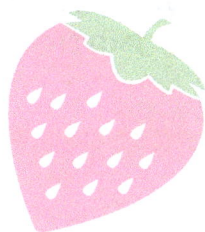

Daily jOurnal

DAY / DATE :

SLEEP
Wake up Time:
Bed Time:
Naps:

ENERGY LEVEL :

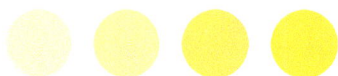

EXERCISE :

Strength	**Flexibility**
Cardio	**Balance**

MY DAILY **EXERCISE** RATED :

TODAY'S WATER
CONSUMPTION :

THREE HEALTHY
FOODS I ATE TODAY:

1

2

3

I conquered this hard thing today:

Strawberry moments:

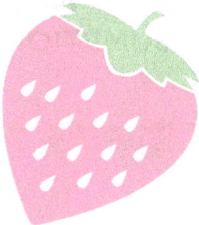

Daily jOurnal

DAY / DATE :

SLEEP
Wake up Time:
Bed Time:
Naps:

ENERGY LEVEL :

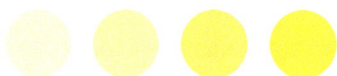

EXERCISE :

Strength	Flexibility

Cardio	Balance

MY DAILY EXERCISE RATED :

THREE HEALTHY FOODS I ATE TODAY:

TODAY'S WATER CONSUMPTION :

1

2

3

I conquered this hard thing today:

Strawberry moments:

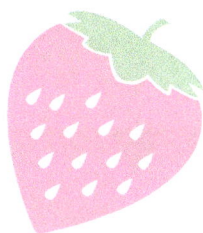

Daily jOurnal

DAY / DATE :

SLEEP
Wake up Time:
Bed Time:
Naps:

ENERGY LEVEL :

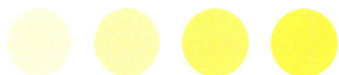

EXERCISE :

Strength	Flexibility
Cardio	Balance

MY DAILY EXERCISE RATED :

THREE HEALTHY
FOODS I ATE TODAY:

TODAY'S WATER
CONSUMPTION :

1

2

3

I conquered this hard thing today:

Strawberry moments:

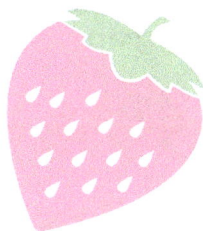

Daily jOurnal

DAY / DATE :

SLEEP
Wake up Time:
Bed Time:
Naps:

ENERGY LEVEL :

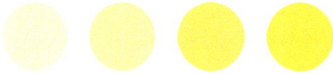

EXERCISE :

Strength	Flexibility

Cardio	Balance

MY DAILY EXERCISE RATED :

TODAY'S WATER
CONSUMPTION :

THREE HEALTHY
FOODS I ATE TODAY:

1

2

3

I conquered this hard thing today:

Strawberry moments:

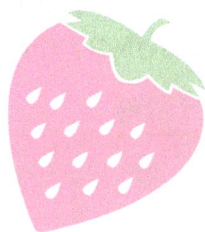

Daily jOurnal

DAY / DATE :

SLEEP
Wake up Time:
Bed Time:
Naps:

ENERGY LEVEL :

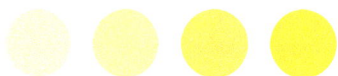

EXERCISE :

Strength	Flexibility
Cardio	Balance

MY DAILY EXERCISE RATED :

TODAY'S WATER
CONSUMPTION :

THREE HEALTHY
FOODS I ATE TODAY:

1

2

3

I conquered this hard thing today:

Strawberry moments:

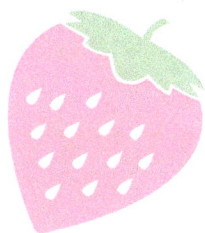

Daily jOurnal

DAY / DATE :

SLEEP
Wake up Time:
Bed Time:
Naps:

ENERGY LEVEL :

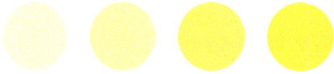

EXERCISE :

Strength	Flexibility

Cardio	Balance

MY DAILY EXERCISE RATED :

THREE HEALTHY
FOODS I ATE TODAY:

TODAY'S WATER
CONSUMPTION :

1

2

3

I conquered this hard thing today:

Strawberry moments:

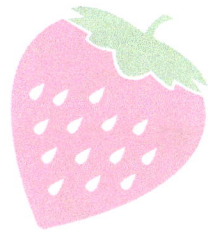

Daily jOurnal

DAY / DATE :

SLEEP
Wake up Time:
Bed Time:
Naps:

ENERGY LEVEL :

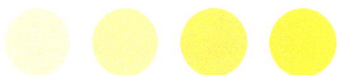

EXERCISE :

Strength	Flexibility
Cardio	Balance

MY DAILY EXERCISE RATED :

TODAY'S WATER
CONSUMPTION :

THREE HEALTHY
FOODS I ATE TODAY:

1

2

3

I conquered this hard thing today:

Strawberry moments:

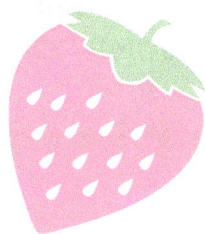

Daily jOurnal

DAY / DATE :

SLEEP
Wake up Time:
Bed Time:
Naps:

ENERGY LEVEL :

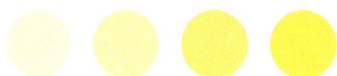

EXERCISE :

Strength	Flexibility

Cardio	Balance

MY DAILY EXERCISE RATED :

THREE HEALTHY
FOODS I ATE TODAY:

TODAY'S WATER
CONSUMPTION :

1

2

3

I conquered this hard thing today:

Strawberry moments:

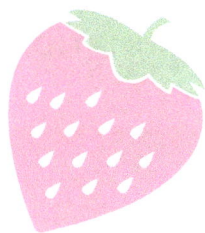

Daily jOurnal

DAY / DATE :

SLEEP
Wake up Time:
Bed Time:
Naps:

ENERGY LEVEL :

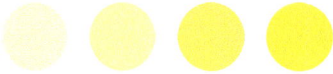

EXERCISE :

Strength	Flexibility

Cardio	Balance

MY DAILY EXERCISE RATED :

TODAY'S WATER
CONSUMPTION :

THREE HEALTHY
FOODS I ATE TODAY:

1

2

3

I conquered this hard thing today:

Strawberry moments:

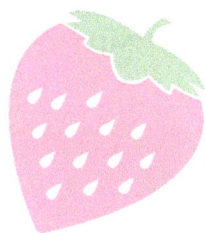

Daily jOurnal

DAY / DATE :

SLEEP
Wake up Time:
Bed Time:
Naps:

ENERGY LEVEL :

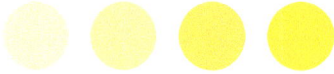

EXERCISE :

Strength	Flexibility
Cardio	Balance

MY DAILY EXERCISE RATED :

THREE HEALTHY
FOODS I ATE TODAY:

1

TODAY'S WATER
CONSUMPTION :

2

3

I conquered this hard thing today:

Strawberry moments:

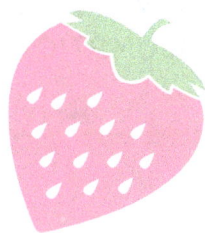

Daily jOurnal

DAY / DATE :

SLEEP
Wake up Time:
Bed Time:
Naps:

ENERGY LEVEL :

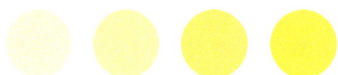

EXERCISE :

Strength	Flexibility

Cardio	Balance

MY DAILY EXERCISE RATED :

THREE HEALTHY
FOODS I ATE TODAY:

1

TODAY'S WATER
CONSUMPTION :

2

3

I conquered this hard thing today:

Strawberry moments:

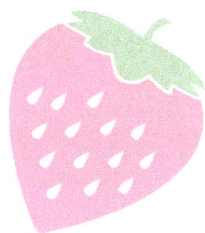

Daily jOurnal

DAY / DATE :

SLEEP
Wake up Time:
Bed Time:
Naps:

ENERGY LEVEL :

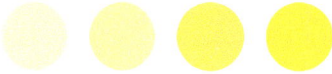

EXERCISE :

Strength	Flexibility
Cardio	Balance

MY DAILY EXERCISE RATED :

THREE HEALTHY
FOODS I ATE TODAY:

1

TODAY'S WATER
CONSUMPTION :

2

3

I conquered this hard thing today:

Strawberry moments:

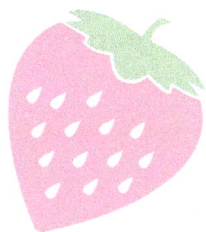

Daily jOurnal

DAY / DATE :

SLEEP
Wake up Time:
Bed Time:
Naps:

ENERGY LEVEL :

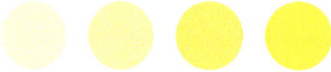

EXERCISE :

Strength	Flexibility

Cardio	Balance

MY DAILY EXERCISE RATED :

THREE HEALTHY
FOODS I ATE TODAY:

1

TODAY'S WATER
CONSUMPTION :

2

3

I conquered this hard thing today:

Strawberry moments:

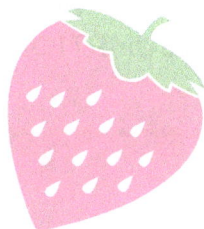

Daily jOurnal

DAY / DATE :

SLEEP
Wake up Time:
Bed Time:
Naps:

ENERGY LEVEL :

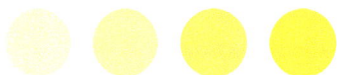

EXERCISE :

Strength	Flexibility

Cardio	Balance

MY DAILY EXERCISE RATED :

TODAY'S WATER
CONSUMPTION :

THREE HEALTHY
FOODS I ATE TODAY:

1

2

3

I conquered this hard thing today:

Strawberry moments:

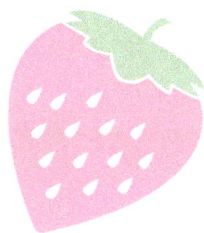

Daily jOurnal

DAY / DATE :

SLEEP
Wake up Time:
Bed Time:
Naps:

ENERGY LEVEL :

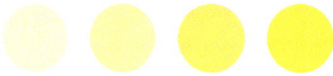

EXERCISE :

Strength	**Flexibility**

Cardio	**Balance**

MY DAILY EXERCISE RATED :

TODAY'S WATER CONSUMPTION :

THREE HEALTHY FOODS I ATE TODAY:

1

2

3

I conquered this hard thing today:

Strawberry moments:

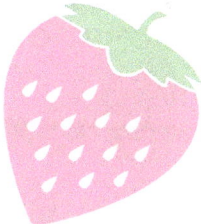

Daily jOurnal

DAY / DATE :

SLEEP
Wake up Time:
Bed Time:
Naps:

ENERGY LEVEL :

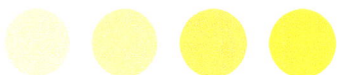

EXERCISE :

Strength

Flexibility

Cardio

Balance

MY DAILY EXERCISE RATED :

TODAY'S WATER
CONSUMPTION :

THREE HEALTHY
FOODS I ATE TODAY:

1

2

3

I conquered this hard thing today:

Strawberry moments:

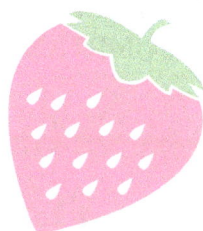

Daily jOurnal

DAY / DATE :

SLEEP
Wake up Time:
Bed Time:
Naps:

ENERGY LEVEL :

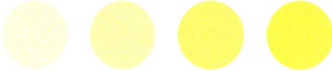

EXERCISE :

Strength	**Flexibility**

Cardio	**Balance**

MY DAILY EXERCISE RATED :

THREE HEALTHY
FOODS I ATE TODAY:

TODAY'S WATER
CONSUMPTION :

1

2

3

I conquered this hard thing today:

Strawberry moments:

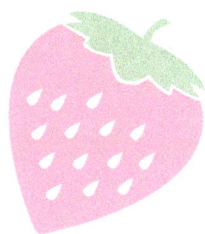

Daily jOurnal

DAY / DATE :

SLEEP
Wake up Time:
Bed Time:
Naps:

ENERGY LEVEL :

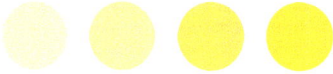

EXERCISE :

Strength	Flexibility

Cardio	Balance

MY DAILY EXERCISE RATED :

TODAY'S WATER CONSUMPTION :

THREE HEALTHY FOODS I ATE TODAY:

1

2

3

I conquered this hard thing today:

Strawberry moments:

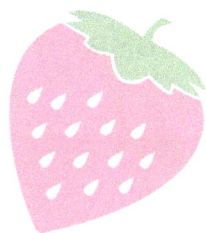

Daily jOurnal

DAY / DATE :

SLEEP
Wake up Time:
Bed Time:
Naps:

ENERGY LEVEL :

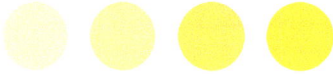

EXERCISE :

Strength	Flexibility
Cardio	Balance

MY DAILY EXERCISE RATED :

THREE HEALTHY
FOODS I ATE TODAY:

1

2

3

TODAY'S WATER
CONSUMPTION :

I conquered this hard thing today:

Strawberry moments:

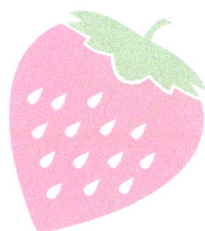

YouR HeAltHy CanCeR CoMebacK

SICK *TO* STRONG

Fitz Koehler, MSESS

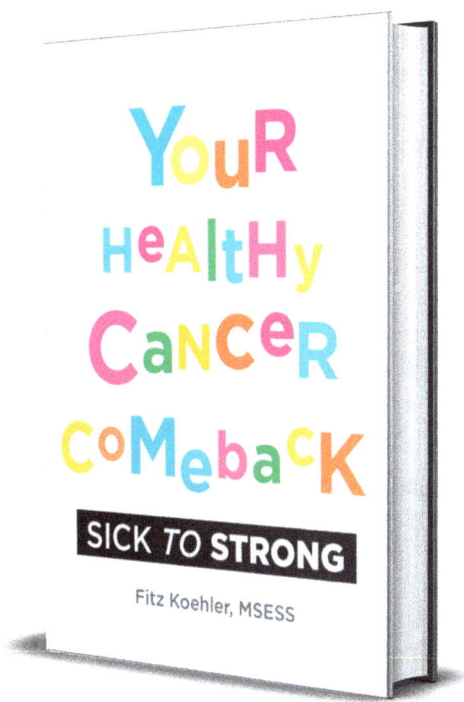

The comprehensive guidebook for cancer patients and survivors eager to maintain and regain strength, stamina, vibrancy, athleticism, and health. Cancers of all types and their treatments can be brutal. Instead of surrendering your health and fitness to this monster, fight back and control the things you can!

Signed copies and bulk orders available at Fitzness.com

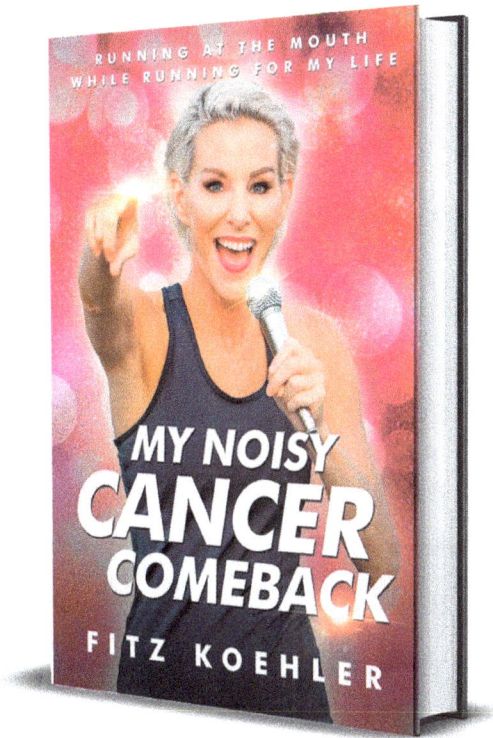

RUNNING AT THE MOUTH WHILE RUNNING FOR MY LIFE

MY NOISY CANCER COMEBACK

FITZ KOEHLER

A funny, dramatic, and honest insight into one very noisy woman's adventures and misadventures while battling cancer. It's the ultimate motivational tool for thriving while surviving! Fitz's story proves that anyone can endure hardships better by utilizing perspective, passion, and positivity.

Available in hardcover, paperback, ebook, and audiobook.

Cancer Comeback 3-pack

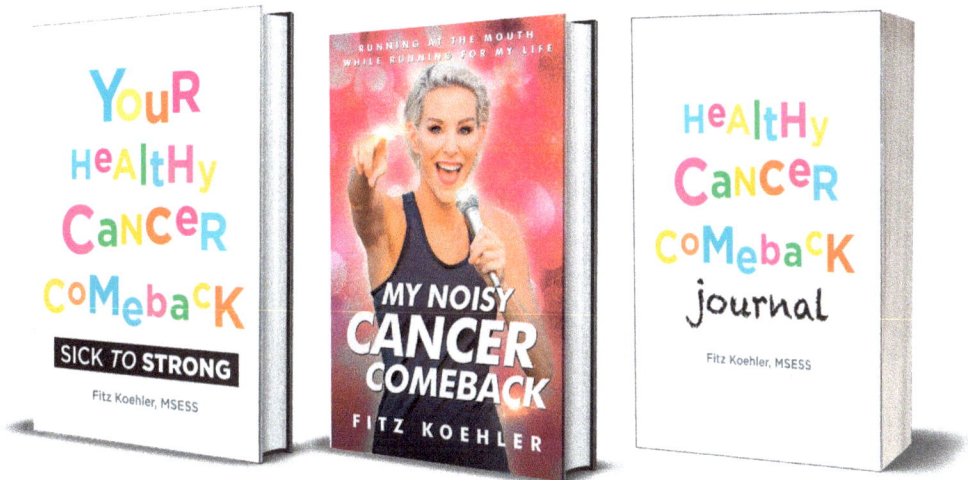

The Cancer Comeback Series is packed with inspiration and information every cancer patient and survivor needs to go from sick to strong! Makes a great gift.

FiTzNeSS.COM

The Fitzness Show
Recipes
Workout Videos
Articles
Training Tips
Fitz's Event Calendar
Books and Online Courses
Cancer Comeback Stories- submit yours!
Inspirational Cancer Comeback Gear
Contact Fitz

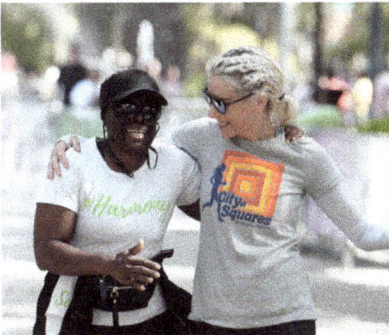

FiTzNeSS.COM

Home Store Contact Meet Fitz Race Announcer Keynote Speaker Fitzness Blog TV/Podcast Appearances Workout Videos The Fitzness Show Fitz vs. Breast Cancer Morning Mile

LIVE
BETTER
AND
LONGER

Motivational Keynote Presentations

Energetic. Entertaining. Compelling.

Book Fitz at Fitzness.com

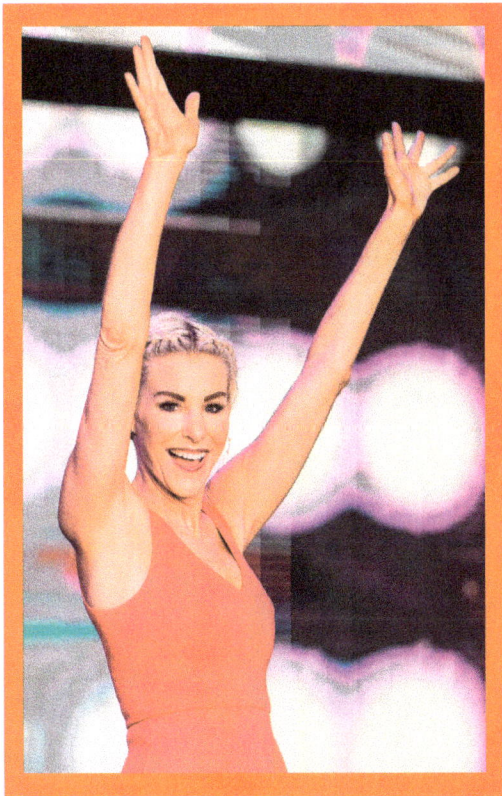

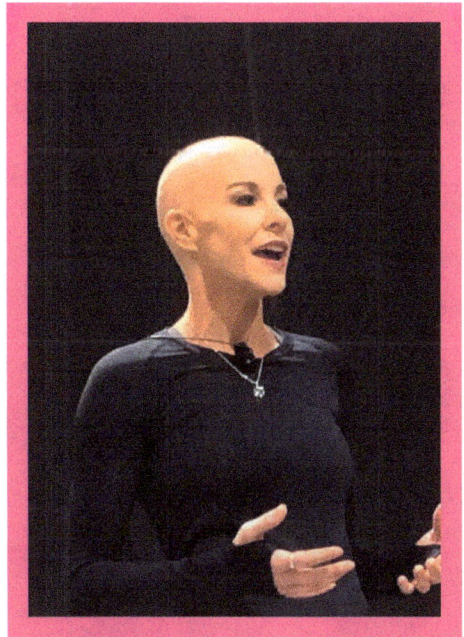

the MORNING MILE®

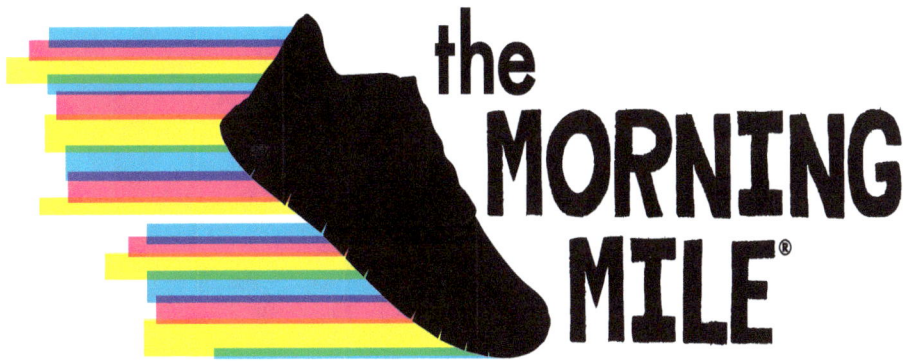

The Morning Mile™ is an easily-implemented before-school walking/running program that gives children a chance to start each day in an active way while enjoying fun, music, and friends. That's EVERY CHILD, EVERY DAY. It's also supported by a wonderful system of rewards, which keeps students highly motivated and frequently congratulated. Inquire to sponsor programs or to get your favorite schools started.

Let's Get More Kids Moving in The Mornings!

MORNINGMILE.COM

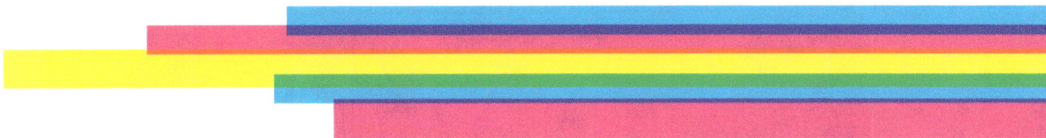

Let's Connect!

FITZNESS on Facebook
@Fitzness on Instagram
@Fitzness on YouTube
Fitz Koehler on Linkedin
Fitzness13 on TikTok
HealthyCancerComeback on Instragram

#FITZNESS
#HealthyCancerComeback

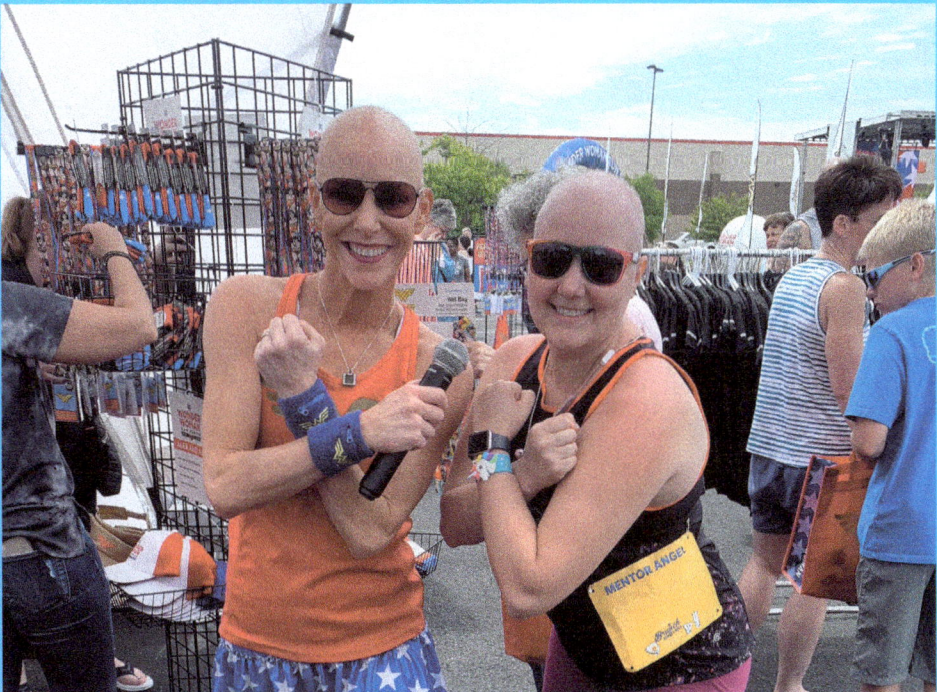

About the Author

Fitz Koehler is among the most prominent and compelling fitness experts and race announcers in America. With a Master's Degree in Exercise and Sport Sciences and decades of experience teaching fitness worldwide, Fitz has helped countless people live better and longer by making fitness understandable, attainable, and fun. As CEO of Fitzness International, she masterfully uses every form of mass media to lead people toward health and athletic adventure.

In 2019, Fitz was diagnosed with breast cancer, and her healthy and athletic body was brutalized by 15 months of chemotherapy, radiation, and surgeries. Instead of shutting down, she turned the volume up on her career. She also strategically orchestrated her own healthy cancer comeback from sick, scrawny, and weak to a strong Boston Marathon finisher. Her memoir *My Noisy Cancer Comeback: Running at the Mouth, While Running for My Life* was released in 2020 and has been a massive source of motivation for those facing hardships of all sorts. Fitz shares inspirational lessons from her cancer-crushing whirlwind in her keynote presentations, convincing global audiences that they "can do hard things," too.

As the voice of the Los Angeles Marathon, Buffalo Marathon, Big Sur Marathon, The Donna Marathon to Finish Breast Cancer,, DC Super Hero Series, and more, Fitz brings big structure, energy, and joy to sports. She has appeared on many national media outlets, hosts a popular podcast, The Fitzness Show, and has performed as a speaker and spokesperson for corporations like Disney®, Oakley®, Tropicana®, and Office Depot®. Fitz's successful school running/walking program, The Morning Mile®, has inspired millions of children, their families, and teachers to get moving in the mornings.

In her free time, Fitz enjoys water sports, strength training, obstacle course races, animals, hugs, sarcasm, getting muddy in her Jeep Wrangler, and travel. She lives in Gainesville, Florida.

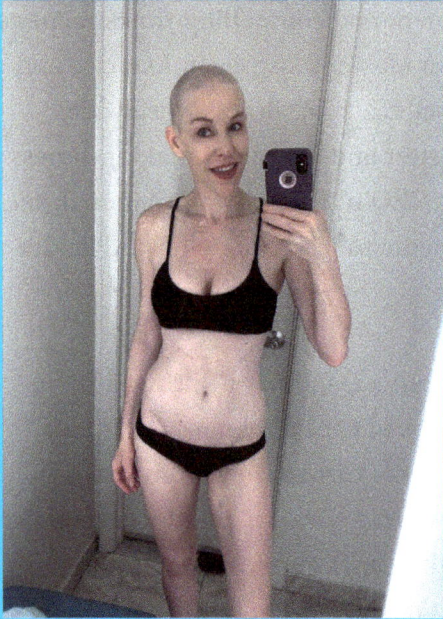

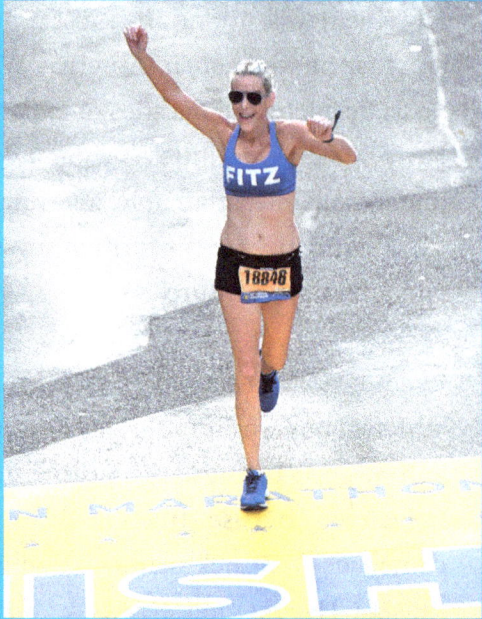

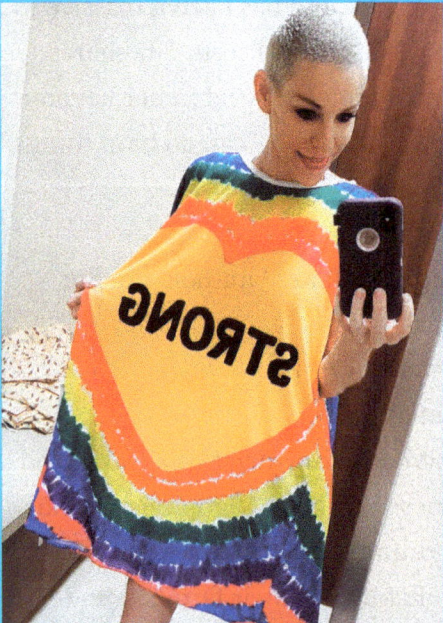

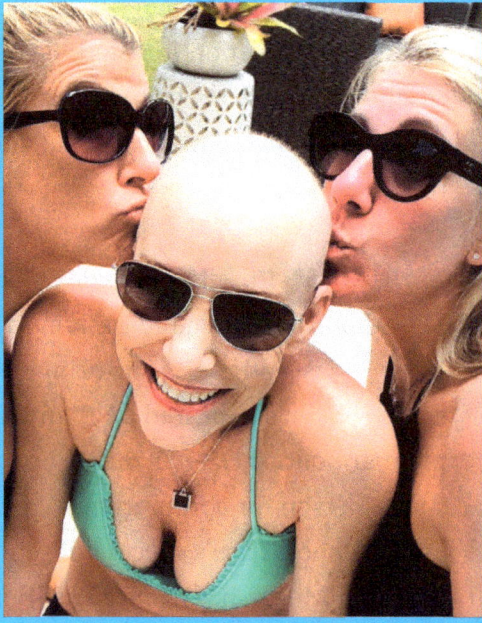

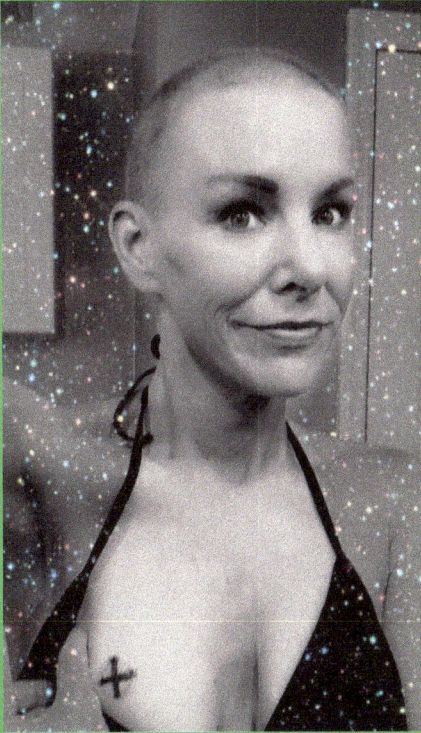

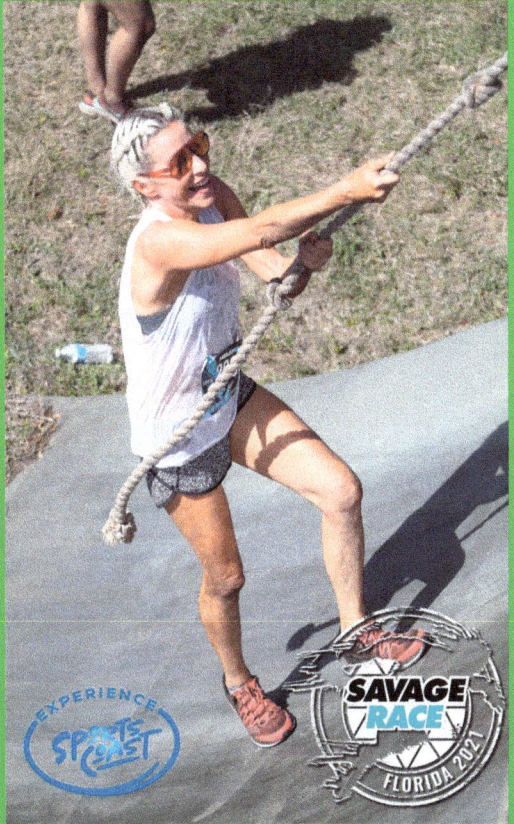

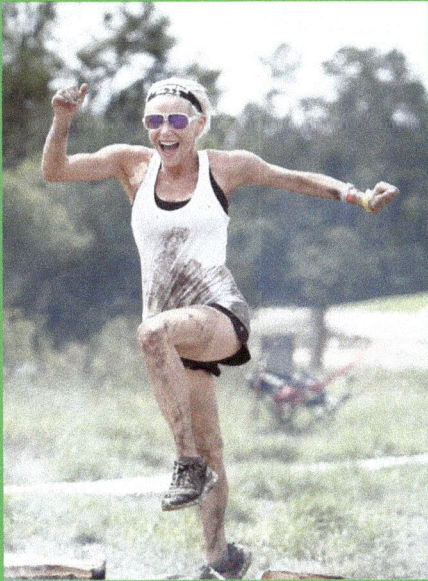

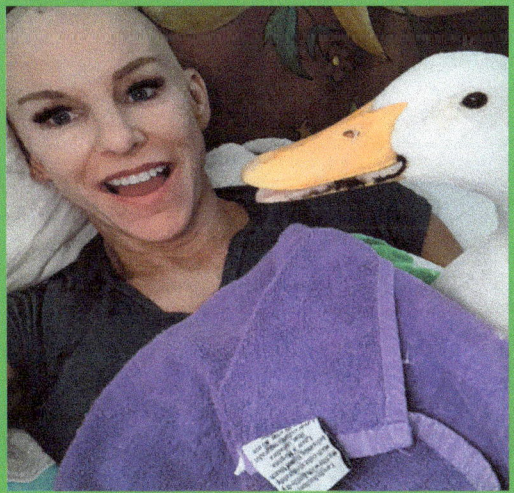

www.ingramcontent.com/pod-product-compliance
Lightning Source LLC
Chambersburg PA
CBHW070613030426

42337CB00020B/3783